SOTHIS PRESS

Sothis Press aims to completely reimagine the public domain book with an emphasis on universal access to captivatingly designed print editions. We believe that technology will enable every single book ever published to be perpetually accessible in beautiful print form. Sothis is beauty in ubiquity.

www.sothis.press
1 Waterhouse Square, London, ECIN 2ST

A Safe, Speedy and Certain Cure for Small-Pox

With Cases Illustrative of Its Efficacy in Every Stage of the Disease, in Preventing Disfigurement, Etc., Etc

Charles Rose

SOTHIS PRESS

ISBN 978-1-83548-652-8

A Safe, Speedy and Certain Cure for Small-Pox
is in the public domain.

This edition is published by
Sothis Press The company
is registered in England and Wales.
The Company Number is 14900389.

A

SAFE, SPEEDY, AND CERTAIN

CURE

FOR

SMALL-POX:

WITH

CASES ILLUSTRATIVE OF ITS EFFICACY IN EVERY STAGE OF THE DISEASE, IN PREVENTING DISFIGUREMENT, Etc., Etc.

"Facts are stubborn things."

Charles Rose

COPYRIGHTED.

WILLIAM ROSE, TRENTON,
WAYNE COUNTY, MICH.

1877.

DETROIT PRINTING COMPANY, 86 WOODWARD AVENUE, DETROIT.

PREFACE.

The world's history has been one of discovery. Age after age has revealed some secret before undivulged; some fact before unknown. A trivial incident has disclosed an economy hitherto undreamt of; a mere accident a mine of wealth hidden for ages. The falling of an apple discovered the law of gravitation; the exhalation from a kettle suggested the steam engine. The gold-fields of Australia and California, trodden over for centuries by rude Aborigines, have not till lately enriched the world with their treasures. Science, with all its enterprise, delving below and peering above, has revealed but a tithe of the world's wonders. The discoveries of future generations might prove as startling to those who live now, as those of our day would be to our ancestors—not the least surprising, perhaps, the new found uses of familiar things. What has already happened may happen again. Gas, steam, electricity—as old as the earth—were each elementarily known to our forefathers. It required, however, an ingenious mind to descry their scientific appropriation; and a skilful hand to apply them to lighting, to locomotion, and to telegraphy.

What is true of science in general, is equally so of medicine in particular. The herb by the wayside, the chemical in the laboratory, the mineral beneath our feet, may yet be found to possess a remedial virtue now unthought of. Diseases, at present regarded as hopelessly remediless, may, by the brighter light of discovery, be easily curable. The order and benificence pervading Creation; the Providential laws, preserving and rectifying, everywhere in operation, point to such a conclusion.

The cooling fruits of summer, while illustrating a wise and kind economy, indicate also the refrigerant uses of acids: hence their remedial employment in fever. In addition to this febrifugal property, they possess, as is well known, an antidotal one also. Every intelligent housewife is aware that vinegar, a vegetable acid, neutralizes the taint of meat—an incipient animal poison. Infectious fevers—

not excepting the variolous or small-pox—are not unfrequently attributable to fetid or ammonical exhalations,* or, as some imagine, to a miasm having an affinity to, and residing in, these exhalations. Experience has shown, that sometimes in typhus fever, an ammoniacal effluvium from the patient is scarcely endurable. Is it unreasonable, therefore, to suppose, that an acid, or acids, may exist, specifically antidotal to the miasm producing these infectious febrile diseases? If it be not, the inference will hardly be an illogical one, that a timely administration of the antidote—as in the case of palpable poisons—might intercept the effect of a deleterious cause. It is surely not beyond the range of probability either, that an antidote to the poison might prove remedial also to the diseased condition resulting from it.

Considerations such as these demand at least a respectful attention to the remedy treated of in this pamphlet: a remedy hitherto regarded perhaps as the offspring of empiricism, but possibly, after all, perfectly harmonious with science.

May not the infrequency of small-pox in the interior of France be attributable to the large amount of tartaric acid in French wines? Judging from the success attending a limited number of experiments with the remedy referred to as a preventive of small-pox, it would appear so.

Whether the theory suggested be a correct one or not, the cases hereafter detailed conclusively show that a remedy exists, specifical to the fever of small-pox in all its stages; and that in ordinary cases, an appropriate administration of the medicine, and a judicious treatment alone are needed, surely and speedily to effect a cure.

Ample details relative to the remedy and treatment will be found in the letter addressed to the medical officers of the small-pox hospital. Further particulars may be gleaned from the cases described.

It may be asked, perhaps, why a discovery so inestimably valuable was not long ago made public. The correspondence on the subject hereafter inserted will furnish a reply. A perusal of it will suggest the difficulty of obtaining even a hearing for a non-professional discovery. Whatever its merits or importance, these, it would appear, in the estimation of some, are far outweighed by other considerations. The value of a discovery, however, does not depend on its professional origin or its official recognition. Let it be judged, as it ought, by its intrinsic worth and its public utility. Medical science has received, ere now, no mean gifts from non-professional hands: it may do so again.

---

* A number of workmen in Southwark were recently employed near a sewer. Five of them failed immediately after with small-pox.

A discovery so important to humanity—a remedy so efficacious in so loathsome and fatal a disease—will doubtless command a generous reception and an attentive consideration from the philanthropic and conscientious medical practitioner.

The advice of friends to patent the remedy has not been adopted. A course more conducive to the general good has been pursued. It has heretofore been offered to Government, to Parliament, to Hospital; it is now published—"A BLESSING TO THE WORLD."

A Letter to the Public.

I wish it to be generally understood that I have no knowledge of any relationship to the discoverer of this most valuable cure for small-pox, though I bear the same family name.

I was raised within a few miles of Dorking, where the author had his discovery in full operation, and have known of several most rapid and wonderful cures by the use of bi-tartrate of potash. As prevention is better than cure, it is a sure preventive, and if taken in time will arrest most all fevers.

When leaving England for this land of my adoption, I brought a copy of this work with me, and I believe it has been the means of preventing a deal of sickness in my own family. I have been in this country now eight years, and have watched with anxiety every time the loathsome disease of small-pox made its appearance around us, expecting that the valuable cure discovered by Mr. Thomas Rose of Dorking, England, might be introduced by some conscientious and philanthropic medical practitioner, but as such has not been the case I feel bound, for humanity's sake (as hundreds are dying annually by that most dreaded of diseases), to publish this work for the benefit of the American people. *The receipt is given as a blessing to the world.*

In concluding my letter to a generous people, I wish it to be understood that I lay no claim to the discovery which is so elaborately described and its mode of treatment made so plain in every stage of the disease, and for all ages, and is made so plain that all might understand it thoroughly, and I trust this pamphlet may find its way into every home in this fair country, there to be stored up as a magazine of wealth, to be relied upon and trusted, should that fell destroyer of life and beauty visit you. Remember, all are liable to its withering blast, and no man is sure to escape ; therefore I ask you to read carefully this pamphlet all through, for it is well to be thoroughly posted with regard to its proper treatment; and remember that it is given as a blessing to the world by the author, and I have determined to assist him in his humane efforts with the small capital at my disposal, in republishing this book at a low price, to enable the poorest person to be in possession of it. And all I ask from a grateful people is to help me by becoming agents for the book, and if every person that is fortunate enough to obtain possession of the receipt will advocate it to their friends, they will perform an act of humane kindness, and very soon the disagreeable practice of vaccination will be pronounced by an outraged and indignant people to be unnecessary. I now conclude with a few lines from the poet:

> **For every evil under the sun**
> **There is a remedy or there is none;**
> **If there is one let us find it,**
> **If there is none never mind it.**

W. ROSE.

Trenton, Wayne County, Michigan.

A SAFE, SPEEDY AND CERTAIN

CURE

FOR

SMALL-POX.

The small-pox has for ages been the pest and dread of nations. At what precise period this loathsome disease first appeared is involved in doubt. Some profess to trace its existence in China and India, long before the time of Hippocrates. It seems clear, however, that in the sixth century it had visited Egypt, and in the tenth our own country. For generations its ravages were appalling. In Europe alone, hundreds of thousands were annually victims to its malignancy; and at one period a fourth of the human race is thought to have borne, in suffering and disfigurement, the effects of its virulence. The treatment of the disease, adopted even in the seventeenth century, must have frightfully increased its fatality. A biographer of Sydenham thus describes it: "The usual mode of dealing with this then fearfully virulent disorder, as with eruptive fevers generally, was as opposite as could well be imagined to the dictates of either nature or common sense. The unhappy patient was loaded with bed-clothes lest one refreshing breeze should fan his burning frame; the curtains were drawn closely round; whilst under the notion of the existence of a peutrescency in the blood, he was all the time plied with a round of stimulant and cordials, to say nothing of the perhaps less potent, but more disgusting ingredients, with which good care was taken that he should be sufficiently charged, described altogether by a nearly contemporary physician, as Venice treacle, Virginian snake-root, zeodary, saffron, volatile salt of hartshorn, powder of viper's flesh, and the like."

Fatal though the small-pox was during the seventeenth and eighteenth centuries, the following statistics show a considerable variation in its virulence;

Marshall's Mortality of Metropolis and Bills of Mortality, in British Museum.

Ten Years.	Average small-pox deaths per 1000.	Ten Years.	Average small-pox deaths per 1000.
1650—1660	48	1730—1740	76
1660—1670	36	1740—1750	77
1670—1680	71	1750—1760	100
1680—1690	73	1760—1770	108
1690—1700	45	1770—1780	98
1700—1710	53	1780—1790	87
1710—1720	81	1790—1800	86
1720—1730	82		

The introduction of inoculation into England took place early in the eighteenth century. High anticipations were raised respecting it. The operation, it is true, was usually advantageous in mitigating personal suffering, and the mortality among those who submitted to it was greatly lessened. Its value to society, however, may be seriously questioned; the mortality from small-pox being in the aggregate—as a reference to the foregoing statistics will show—by no means diminished. The dissemination of the disease and the danger of contamination, counterbalanced in disadvantage the benefit of modification.

The discovery of vaccination was hailed with delight. Its discoverer alleged that it was "attended with the singularly beneficial effect of rendering the person so inoculated perfectly secure from the infection of small-pox."

The brightest hopes were cherished that henceforth the fell destroyer of the human race would exist no more. Parliament in gratitude for so hopeful a boon voted to Dr. Jenner, in 1802, £10,000, and in 1807, £20,000 more. The high expectations once entertained respecting vaccination have failed however to be realized. More than half a century has passed away since its introduction, yet the greatest diversity of opinion still prevails respecting it. Its nature;* the day of its maturity; the eligibility of its directness from the cow; its deterioration by transmission; the extent and duration of its protective power; the propriety of its re-performance; the question as to its possessing a prophylactic virtue at all;† its effect upon the general health; the transmission of other diseases by the operation‡ are each and all subjects of keen discussion. While theorists contend, facts reveal the truth. The Registrar General's weekly return, January 10th, 1863, reports that "a boy, aged one year, died of scrofula, caused by impure vaccination." The excellent Sir Culling Eardley has since fallen a victim to re-vaccination. The *Medical Times* of

***Equine lymph*, or in less fine and homely phrase "the grease" from horses' heels, is said to be similar in nature to vaccine. The employment of the former is recommended in the Report of the Committee of the Medical Association for 1859.

†The Registrar General's returns for the weeks ending June 20th, June 27th, July 4th, July 11th, and July 18th, report in the aggregate the occurrence of 42 deaths from small-pox after vaccination.

‡Referring to this question, M. Ricord, a high medical authority, in a lecture recently delivered by him at the Hotel Dieu, Paris, said: "If ever the transmission of disease with vaccine lymph is clearly demonstrated, *vaccination must be altogether discontinued*, for, in the present state of science, we are in possession of no criterion which may permit the conscientious practitioner to assert that the lymph he vaccinates with is perfectly free from admixture with tainted blood.

May 30th last, records the decease of a lady from the same cause.* The great increase of infant mortality, amounting in the aggregate to 254,000 deaths in the seven years immediately succeeding the passing of the compulsory vaccination act, is ominously suggestive. The fact is equally so that this mortality is to a considerable extent proportionate to the vaccinations performed.† "Does vaccination prevent small-pox?" asks "C. T. P.," a medical practitioner, in a letter to the *Daily Telegraph* of May 18th, 1863. "As at present performed it appears doubtful, seeing that 81 per cent. of the Small-pox Hospital patients, recently admitted, were found to have been vaccinated; and already in the first three months of the present year, between forty and fifty have died who had been vaccinated." "These facts," continues the same writer, "are serious, and there is no wonder that the public—rich and poor alike—are ever asking the question, 'What is the use of vaccination?' and thousands are disinclined to run the risk of being impregnated with diseases which may be conveyed into their system by vaccine lymph."‡

Small-pox, notwithstanding the general prevalence of vaccination, —more general, perhaps, than at any previous period,—notwithstanding the enforcement of vaccination by an un-English law, and an

---

* This lady was revaccinated on the 14th of May, from "good matter from the vesicle of a healthy child." On the following morning very singular symptoms had set in; the arm was much swollen, and had a dark purplish hue, much resembling bullock's liver, the punctures nearly invisible, and the whole region of the operation presenting the appearance of having been bitten by a venomous reptile. Remedies were applied, but the patient rapidly grew worse; other professional advice was necessary, and Dr. Bridge, of Argyll-place, Mr. Tatum, of St. George's Hospital, and Dr. MacKenna, of Great Marlborough-street, attended; but the symptoms entirely baffled their skill and experience, and the patient died at midnight of the 18th, of (as agreed by the gentlemen named) phlegmonous [inflammatory] erysipelas.—*Letter of Mr. J. W. Wells, Assistant-Surgeon, of many years' practice.*

† On March 7th, 1859, Lord Granville, the President of the Privy Council, stated to the House of Lords, that the vaccinations performed bore certain proportions to the births in a series of years. The Right Hon, R. Lowe, in his speech to the House of Commons, on the 10th of J y, 1861, gave the statistics of infant mortality for eight years. The following is a tabular result of such statements:

Date.			Proportion of Vaccinations to Births.			Deaths from all causes under one year.
1853*	..	..	33 per cent.	..	..	318,000
1854	..	..	65 "	..	..	408,000
1855	..	..	56 "	..	..	354,000
1856	..	..	54 "	..	..	350,000
1857	..	..	52 "	..	..	338,000
1858	..	..	— "	..	..	341,000
1859	..	..	— "	..	..	335,000
1860	..	..	— "	..	..	354,000

* Compulsory Vaccination Act passed 20th of August.

‡ The concluding portion of this gentleman's letter is too interesting and important not to be given: "The people are taxed, and so far from small-pox being prevented, there is not the slightest doubt that filthy diseases have been conveyed from child to child, while the vaccine lymph has been held in abeyance. Jenner maintained that vaccination was preventive for life. Now, seeing that vaccination is a failure, septennial vaccination is proposed. That which you call 'stupid mistrust' on the part of the public, is well-founded doubt. I have had considerable experience, in my professional capacity, of small-pox, and have just attended a lady, who had been vaccinated for confluent small-pox, in its most severe form. There is no doubt, sir, that public faith in vaccination is shaken, and the remedy is, not to enforce it upon an unwilling people, but to appoint a Royal Commission to inquire into the whole subject. In the meantime, let there be provision for the reception of small-pox cases, in an hospital, in the South of London, and another at the East-end of London, near those foul and fetid hovels where, as you properly remark, small-pox is generated. Did your space permit a longer letter, I could produce much startling evidence to show that small-pox has never been diminished by vaccination. As you say, 'In the present century, we have so long enjoyed a comparative immunity, that we have reposed in fancied security.' Small-pox, as a direful malady, had faded away in this country before vaccinaticn was fashionable. Statistics which I could furnish prove this fact."

annual expenditure in England and Wales alone, from private sources and public funds, of probably £200,000 or £250,000 for its performance,—notwithstanding the great improvement in the treatment of small-pox and the attention of late years to sanitary reform,*—notwithstanding this despotic legislation—this vast expenditure—this amelioration in treatment, small-pox still yearly slays its hundreds and its thousands. Of this, the following statistics, courteously furnished by the Registrar General, are lamentably illustrative :—

Deaths from Small-pox in England and Wales. 1851–61, (including London).

1851	6,997
1852	7,320
1853	3,151
1854	2,808
1855	2,525
1856	2,277
1857	3,936
1858	6,460
1859	3,848
1860	2,749
1861	1,320
1862 not at present known.	
Mortality in 11 years, ...	43,391

Deaths from Small-pox in England and Wales in 1861, (including London).

All ages, ...	1,320
Under 1 year, ...	330
1 year, ...	153
2 “	98
3 “	73
4 “	69
Under 5 years, ...	723
5 years, ...	140
10 “	60
15 “	72
20 “	89
25 “	100
35 “	62
45 “	51
55 “	17
65 “	3
75 “	1
85 “	2
95 and upwards, ...	—

* Both means highly contributory to a diminution of the fatality of small-pox, but appropriated to the enhancement of vaccination.

DEATHS FROM SMALL-POX IN LONDON FROM 1850 TO 1862 (BOTH INCLUSIVE.)

1850	498
1851	1,066
1852	1,166
1853	217
1854	676
1855	1,024
1856	522
1857	154
1858	247
1859	1,156
1860	877
1861	215
1862	345
Mortality in 13 years, ...	8,163

DEATHS IN THE SMALL-POX HOSPITAL, REGISTERED IN THE FIFTY-TWO WEEKS ENDING SATURDAY, 27TH DECEMBER, 1862.

Males, ...	36
Females, ...	20
Total, ...	56

DEATHS FROM SMALL-POX, IN LONDON, IN THE QUARTER ENDING—

April 2, 1859.	March 31, 1860.	March 30, 1861.	March 29, 1862.	MARCH 28, 1863.				
				Under 20 years.	20 and under 40.	40 and under 50.	60 and upwards.	Total.
				296	103	23	None.	
201	464	73	37					422

DEATHS FROM SMALL-POX, IN LONDON, REGISTERED IN THE EIGHTEENTH WEEK OF EACH OF THE FOLLOWING YEARS.

May 7, 1853.	May 6, 1854.	May 5, 1855.	May 3, 1856.	May 9, 1857.	May 8, 1858.	May 7, 1859.	May 5, 1860.	May 4, 1861.	May 3, 1862.	May 2, 1863.
1	12	15	8	2	3	26	18	8	2	68

DEATHS FROM SMALL-POX. IN LONDON, REGISTERED IN THE WEEKS ENDING RESPECTIVELY—

1863—Deaths.	1863—Deaths.	1863—Deaths.	1863—Deaths.	1863—Deaths.	1863—Deaths.
Jan. 3...35	Feb. 7...28	Mar. 7...42	Apr. 4...45	May 2...68	June 6...56
" 10...24	" 14...23	" 14...47	" 11...68	" 9...71	" 13...43
" 17...21	" 21...25	" 21...45	" 18...62	" 16...61	" 20...64
" 24...17	" 28...42	" 28...34	" 25...65	" 23...68	" 27...49
" 31...39	....	....	....	" 30...68	....

Total number of deaths returned during the present year, to June 27, 1,210.

It will thus be seen that no fewer than 43,391 persons were victims to small-pox in England and Wales in eleven years; that of those who died from the disease in 1861, more than half were under five years of age;* and that during the portion of the present year already expired, more than 1,200 have died of it in London alone.

Humanity, groaning and writhing under so loathsome a disease—Affection, with tears, mourning her bereavements—Philanthropy, wistfully gazing heavenward for relief, each imploringly ask, Is there nought in Creation to allaviate this suffering, and to avert this mortality? There is. In the Providence of God a remedy has been discovered, a remedy so simple as to be perfectly innocuous, and so efficacious, as in any stage of this dreaded disease to be uniformly effectual. THREE THOUSAND CASES of small-pox cured by the Bitartrate of Potash—Cream of Tartar—attest its virtues. Taken at the first stage of the disease, it at once arrests the fever and restores the patient. Administered when the sufferer, burning, swollen, livid, delirious, apparently ready to die, it has given relief and effected a cure.

The discovery of the specified virtues of cream of tartar in small-pox, was made by the writer's father, the late Mr. T. Rose, of Dorking, in 1826. "Thinking"—to use his own words—"Cream of Tartar a good thing for fever," he applied it to the cure of small-pox. The experiment was highly successful. Shortly after this discovery, Mr. Rose tested the virtues of the specific in the cases of 1,000 persons, inoculated by himself. Legal proceedings were thereupon instituted against him. A trial at Kingston, toward the close of 1827, terminated, however, in his favor, and a popular demonstration in January, 1828, took place in consequence. During the 20 years succeeding this period, the opportunities for still further trying the efficacy of the remedy were both frequent and numerous. In August, 1848, Mr. Rose, by the advice of the late W. J. Denison, Esq., long the parliamentary representative of the county, and afterwards of the Western division of Surrey, addressed a letter, respecting this discovery, to Sir George Grey, Her Majesty's Secretary of State for the Home Department. It was thought, and not unreasonably, perhaps, that a boon so invaluable to the nation, deserved a nation's reward. An offer was made, therefore, to disclose the discovery, on a guarantee of remuneration. Mr. Denison, who had an intimate acquaintance with the success of the remedy, not only allowed the use of his name as a referee, but kindly exercised his good offices also, in forwarding the communication.

The following is the letter referred to:

AUGUST, 1848.

SIR—I am induced, at the repeated solicitation of friends, to acquaint you that I am in possession of an effectual remedy for the Small-pox, which I now offer to make public on a satisfactory remuneration being given to me.

I have used the remedy referred to, for the last 20 years, in the cases of patients of various ages, in every stage of the disease, and under the most desperate circumstances; sometimes after being given up by members of the

* The Compulsory Vaccination Act requires, with certain special exceptions, under a penalty not exceeding twenty shillings, the Vaccination, within four months after its birth, of every child born in England and Wales since August 1st, 1853.

medical profession, at whose request I have subsequently attended the patient, and have found it perfectly efficacious, not only in the prevention of death, but in so destroying the virulent character of the disease, as to render it comparatively harmless, even to the prevention of disfigurement from its effects.

The cases of more than 3,000 persons, in and around this neighborhood, have during the time named been treated with perfect success, solely by the means I have employed. Out of the large number who have been under my care, but one fatal case has occurred, that of a child, whose death (as its medical attendant is willing to certify) was not caused by one, but by a complication of diseases. I feel it right to state that about 1,000 of the number specified were inoculated by myself previous to the passing of the law for its prohibition. I beg to express my willingness to demonstrate the efficacious nature of the remedy employed, by its effects on a reasonable number of patients in any part of the kingdom, on receiving a guarantee of remuneration on satisfactory success.

I have been an inhabitant of this town for the last 40 years, and long known to W. J. Denison, Esq., M. P., who has kindly consented to give his attestation to the respectability of my character. If requisite, I can also refer you with confidence to other gentlemen of the neighborhood.

I shall be honored by your favoring me with an interview, when I should be able to explain the matter more fully, and, I trust, to your satisfaction.

Waiting your reply, I have the honor to be, sir, your most obedient and humble servant, THOMAS ROSE.

To Sir George Grey, Bart., Secretary of State for the Home Department.

A reply to this communication, from the Home Secretary, dated the 19th of the same month, briefly informed Mr. Denison that Mr. Rose's letter had been transmitted to the Council Office, as the subject belonged to that department. Nothing further, however, was heard of the matter.

The appointment of Sir Benjamin Hall to the General Board of Health presidency was regarded with hope. The subjoined letter was therefore addressed to him:

DORKING, June 14th, 1854.

SIR—I beg most respectfully to enclose for your perusal, a copy of a letter addressed some time since to Sir George Grey, Bart., together with his reply to the late W. J. Denison, Esq.

Permit me also to submit the same subject to your considerate attention.

Since the date of the enclosed letter, the efficacy of my remedy for small-pox has been repeatedly and uniformly demonstrated, in some instances as recently as the last few weeks.

I deem it right at once and frankly to state that I am not a member of the medical profession.

I am willing, as far as my present health will permit, to adhere to the conditions proposed in my letter to Sir George Grey, and should be happy in giving a fuller explanation by an interview.

Awaiting your reply, I am, sir, your most obedient servant,

THOMAS ROSE.

To Sir Benjamin Hall, Bart., President of the General Board of Health.

The letter from Sir G. Grey to Mr. Denison was enclosed with this communication, but the receipt of the latter was not even acknowledged, and the former never returned.

All hope of attention in the official quarters applied to thus being gone, Mr. Rose, in the following spring, addressed a petition to Parliament. In this petition the secret of the discovery was disclosed. This step was taken on the recommendation of the late T. S. Duncombe, Esq., the representative of Finsbury.

The petition was presented to the House of Commons on the 31st of March. The following is a copy:

To the Honorable the Commons of Great Britain and Ireland, in Parliament assembled. The humble Petition of Thomas Rose, of West Street, Dorking, in the County of Surrey, sheweth:

That your Petitioner in the year 1826, discovered Cream of Tartar to be a specific for the fever of small-pox, and has since found the remedial action of the same to be assisted by Rhubarb.

That your petitioner, from the said year to the present time, has tested the virtue of his discovery in the cases of considerably more than 3000 persons, about 1000 of whom were inoculated by your petitioner before its legal prohibition, and the remainder having imbibed small-pox by infection.

That your petitioner has proved the uniform efficacy of his remedy in every stage of small-pox; in many instances when those under its influence had been given over by their medical attendant.

That of the vast number of those who have been under the treatment of your petitioner, but one—a child suffering from whooping cough at the same time—has fallen a victim to small-pox, and that therefore your petitioner has the strongest reason to believe that the fatality which too frequently results from small-pox might by the employment of this remedy be averted.

That by administering the said specific on the first development of small-pox, and the adoption of a mode of treatment which your petitioner is about to publish, he has invariably found that the fever is speedily allayed, the patient soon restored to health, and disfigurement prevented.

That your petitioner respectfully submits, that by the prompt administration of his specific, and the adoption of his mode of treatment, they become thereby not only the means of cure, but of prevention also, inasmuch as the probability of infection to others is greatly diminished, if not entirely removed.

That your petitioner has not employed his remedy professionally, nor for any fee, and hereby makes it known to your Honorable House for the general good, believing, as he does, that its publication will prove a blessing to the world.

Wherefore your petitioner humbly prays your Honorable House to take such steps as in its wisdom it may see fit, to test and to publish the virtue of the said remedy; and specially, that this his petition may be printed with the votes of your Honorable House. And your petitioner, as in duty bound, will ever pray.

(Signed) THOMAS ROSE.

The hopes raised by the presentation of this important petition were doomed to disappointment. Its prayer was not complied with. The following notice of it, however, was given in the Eighteenth Report of the Select Committee on Public Petitions (March 31st, 1856):

SMALL-POX.—For inquiry as to invention. 6716 March 31. Thomas Rose, of West street, Dorking, in the County of Surrey, (Mr. Henry Drummond ......1.

The petitioner states that in 1826, he discovered Cream of Tartar to be a specific for the fever of small-pox, and has since found the remedial action of the same to be assisted by Rhubarb; he has tested his remedy unprofessionally, and without fee, in upwards of 3000 cases, and proved its efficacy in every stage of that disease, only one person of all those cases, a child suffering from whooping cough, having fallen a victim; he considers that the publication of such remedy would prove a general blessing, and prays the House to adopt measures for testing and publishing the same, and also that his petition may be printed with the votes.

A second reference to the remedy, as follows, is to be found in the Forty-sixth Report of the Select Committee on Public Petitions (16-19th June, 1856):

VACCINATION.—For inquiry. 12,775. June 19. Edward and Hannah Batchelor, inhabitants of Dorking, in the County of Surrey,* (Dr. Mitchell).....2.

The petitioners state that they are convinced that vaccination is not a preventive of small-pox ; that pernicious effects sometimes result from vaccination; and that cream of tartar, assisted by rhubarb, is a specific for that disease; and they pray the House not to sanction an extension of compulsory vaccination, but to direct an investigation into the said remedy.

The decease of Mr. Rose occurred in July, 1858, and in the following year the writer obtained insertion of a paragraph relative to the remedy, in the *West Surrey Times*. A copy of this paragraph was forwarded to the leading metropolitan and provincial journals. Editorial—perhaps Esculapian—censorship consigned it however in the great majority of instances, to the waste basket.

The severe small-pox epidemic in the metropolis during the present year (1863), called again for action.

A petition was therefore addressed by the writer to the House of Commons. The statements as to the discovery and success of the specific, contained in the late Mr. Rose's petition, were recapitulated, and the prayer repeated, that the House would "take such steps as in its wisdom it might see fit, to test and publish the virtues of the said remedy." The petition was presented on the 4th of May, by J. I. Briscoe, M. P. for West Surrey. Some technical objection to its being printed existing, Mr. Briscoe vainly attempted to obtain for it a place with the votes of the House. The *West Surrey Times* of May 2d anticipated its presentation by inserting the petition *in extenso*, and by a leading article upon it. Referring to the supposed remedy for small-pox, the *Sarracena Purpurea*†, the article referred to went on to remark—"This vegetable product may, for ought we know, possess all the remedial virtue ascribed to it; but why, it may be asked, travel so far distant for a little known remedy, when one familiar to us all exists at home? If what is stated in a petition, which we print under our Dorking heading, be authentic, the pure Bi-tartrate of Potash, popularly known as Cream of Tartar, equals, if not surpasses, in its antidotal efficacy, any other remedy for small-pox. As will be seen by a perusal of the petition referred to, the discoverer of this alleged specific—Mr. T. Rose, of Dorking—some two or three years before his decease, communicated his discovery to Parliament. No notice, however, was taken of his petition, and he went to his grave with the simple reward of having performed a duty. The fearful mortality from small-pox now prevailing is surely enough to incite attention to what is alleged to be so efficacious a remedy. If in the hands of its unprofessional discoverer, its success was so remarkable, what might it not be made to effect by the application of medical science and skill? The public health and safety, menaced by the presence of a fatal epidemic, demand for it at least a respectful consideration and an impartial trial."

* Some of the petitioners' children were afflicted with eruptions through vaccination, and caught the small-pox shortly after the operation. They were speenily cured by Mr. Rose's remedy. Hence the petition.

† It has been since stated that the *Sarracenia* "has failed entirely to do any good."

Two days only were allowed to elapse before a copy of the article alluded to, and of the writer's petition, were enclosed to the Privy Council. The subjoined letter was at the same time addressed to their Lordships:

DORKING, May 4th, 1863.

MY LORDS—I beg leave most respectfully to solicit your attention to the specific for Small-pox, referred to in the petition and article enclosed.

Permit me, my Lords, to express my willingness, freely and unconditionally, to lay before your Lordships all the details in my possession relative to the remedy referred to, and to the mode of treatment so successfully adopted by my late father, for the cure of small-pox.

Allow me, my Lords, to indulge the hope that, at the present time, when the prevalence of small-pox in the metropolis is so extensive, and the mortality from it so lamentably great, a remedy so simple, so harmless, so efficacious, and so universally applicable, may receive your Lordships' prompt and favorable consideration.

Awaiting your Lordships' commands, I beg to subscribe myself, your Lordships' obedient servant, CHARLES ROSE.

To the Right Honorable, the Lords of Her Majesty's Privy Council.

The following reply to this communication was afterwards received:

MEDICAL DEPARTMENT OF THE PRIVY COUNCIL OFFICE,
May 11th, 1863.

SIR—I am directed by the Lords of her Majesty's Council to acknowledge the receipt of your letter of May 4th, informing their Lordships that you believe yourself to be possessed of a specific for the successful treatment of small-pox, and enclosing (as an extract from the West Surrey Times) the copy of a petition, which you have addressed to the House of Commons, as well as some printed remarks on the same subject. And I am to state to you that their Lordships (according to their usual method of dealing with such communications) have transmitted your enclosuie to the Small-pox Hospital.

I am, sir, your obedient servant,

JOHN SIMON.

Charles Rose, Esq., Dorking.

A letter, as follows, detailing the remedy and treatment, was then addressed to the Small-pox Hospital:

DORKING, May 13th, 1863.

GENTLEMEN—I beg to inform you that my late father having discovered the purified Bi-tartrate of Potash to be a specific for the Variolous Fever, and having successfully tested the efficacy of his discovery in 3,000 cases of Small-pox, I felt it a duty, specially during the prevalence of this epidemic in the metropolis, to communicate this information to the Lords of her Majesty's Privy Council.

As in a reply to my communication, received yesterday, it is stated that their Lordships (according to their usual method of dealing with such communications) have transmitted my enclosure to the Small-pox Hospital; permit me to lay before you the details relative to the remedy referred to, and to the treatment of small-pox, so successfully adopted.

Shortly after the discovery alluded to was made, its uniform efficacy was proved in the cases of more than 1,000 persons, inoculated by my late father. Many cases of natural small-pox were treated cotemporaneously, with unvarying success. Some of these cases were of a most desperate character, and had been given over as hopeless, by the medical attendant. In every instance, however, soon after the administration of the specific, an improvement was perceptible, and a cure happily effected. A few years afterwards an unsuccessful case occurred, that of a child, who suffered from whooping-cough simultaneously with the small pox. In the course of my father's great experience in the treatment of small-pox, and his numerous opportunities of observation, he resolved on trying the efficacy of his remedy in the earliest stage of the eruption. The experiment resulted in the most gratifying success. It was uniformly discovered that by administering it at this stage of the disease, the fever was at once subdued, the eruption arrested, and suppuration prevented. It was no less gratifying to find that no injurious result was observable from thus promptly checking the disease. The experience of years, in the cases of persons thus treated, has only served to confirm this statement.

In the earlier years of his treatment of small-pox, my father gave simply the cream of tartar dissolved in water, and administered cold. In cases where the patient was too ill to swallow a draught, it was given with a feather applied to his lips. Rhubarb was, however, afterwards administered in conjunction.

The following are the proportions:

Cream of Tartar, ¾ ounce.
Rhubarb, 12 grains.
Water, 1 pint.

Half a pint of the medicine was given to an adult, in the early-stage cases, on the first appearance of the eruption, and the same quantity repeated as a dose, in three or four hours afterwards. It is worthy of remark, however, that in recent instances, only one of the doses indicated, or the same quantity (half a pint) administered in two doses, has been given, with equal benefit.* The uniform result from administering the medicine at any subsequent stage of the disease has been the speedy subjugation of the fever and a remarkably rapid cure of the patient. The time occupied, however, in perfecting recovery is to some extent dependent on the severity of the case and the stage attained by the disease. In cases characterized by delirium, great benefit has been obtained by applying a bottle of hot water to the feet. Particular attention has been paid to the ventilation of the patient's apartment; to administering all beverages cold; and to his abstaining from everything promotive of fever. Pastry has been prohibited. Meat, also, except in cases when excessive suppuration has so exhausted the patient as to render nutriment of that nature indispensable. These restrictions, however, refer chiefly to the more advanced cases. In the earlier ones they have been found unnecessary. The later-stage patient has been directed to get up and have his clothes put on as soon as possible. An out-door airing at the earliest period practicable has been invariably recommended. But little pitting has resulted, even in the severe cases, under this treatment; and, as will be readily imagined, none in those promptly attended to. In a considerable number of cases, some of the worst character, the patients had been previously vaccinated.

The great importance of arresting the disease at the earliest stage, and thus, in a great degree, preventing its propagation, must be apparent.

I have thus endeavored, gentlemen, to give you the details both as to my father's remedy and treatment. Should you desire further information, and I be able to give it, it will give me pleasure to furnish it.

I have thought it desirable to note down a few of the cases for publication. Some of these were treated by my father; others have come under my own observation. They extend over a period of seven years, the most recent occurring during the present week.

It has given me satisfaction to receive lately the testimony of two members of the medical profession, in this locality, to the efficacy of the specific referred to.

At the request of my brother-in-law, the late G. Tranter, Esq., for many years Superintendent Surgeon of the Malwa Contingent, Mehidpoor, Central India, the remedy and treatment herein detailed were forwarded to him. His lamentable death, however, a few weeks after its receipt, prevented the realization of his intention to test them.

* Subsequent experience has shown that, in severe cases especially, a half-pint dose should be administered.

I need scarcely state that, after the lengthened experience of my father in the success of his discovery, combined with the professional testimony alluded to, and my own observation, I have the strongest confidence in its remedial virtues.

It is now more than fourteen years since it was first submitted to the attention of Government, and, judging from the oft-repeated proofs of its efficacy, both previously and subsequently, there is every reason to believe that, had it been then adopted, the frightful mortality from small-pox, which has since occurred, might have been almost entirely, if not wholly averted.

It would be ungenerous, not to say unjust, to suppose, seeing it has now been transmitted to you by her Majesty's Privy Council, that it will not receive from you an immediate and impartial trial. I shall await with interest, and confidence, to hear the result.

Reserving the right of publishing, with other correspondence in my possession, this communication, and any other I may receive from or make to you on this subject.

I beg to subscribe myself, gentlemen, yours most respectfully,

CHARLES ROSE.

The Medical Officers of the Small-pox Hospital.

P. S.—Since writing the above I have heard, with the highest gratification, of the demonstrated efficacy of the specific at a period prior to the appearance of the eruption. The important question now arises whether, if administered to individuals exposed to small-pox, it might not prove an invaluable prophylactic. This is being tested.

The receipt of this communication was acknowledged by the following letter:

SMALL-POX AND VACCINATION HOSPITAL,
HIGHGATE-HILL, UPPER HOLLOWAY, N.,
LONDON, May 18th, 1863.

SIR—I beg to acknowledge the receipt of your communication respecting the use of cream of tartar in small-pox.

It shall have an impartial trial. I shall test it as I did lately the *Sarracenia*, by selecting the severe cases admitted in the early stage, that have never been vaccinated.

I will inform you of the result of the trial.

I remain, sir, your obedient servant,

J. F. MARSON, Surgeon.

Charles Rose, Esq.

The contents of the subjoined letter will explain the reasons for its communication:

DORKING, May 26th, 1863.

MY LORDS—I beg most respectfully to acknowledge the receipt of a letter from the Medical Officer of your most Honorable Council, in reply to my communication to your Lordships relative to my late father's specific for small-pox.

I have the honor to state, also, that, being informed your Lordships had transmitted my communication to the Small-pox Hospital, I addressed a letter, on the 13th inst., to the medical officers of that institution, fully detailing the remedy referred to, and the treatment adopted in conjunction with its administration. In a reply to this letter, from the resident surgeon of the hospital, I am apprised that an impartial trial shall be given to the specific, and the result communicated.

Permit me, my Lords, to acquaint you that, since addressing my former communication to your Most Honorable Council, I have ascertained the interesting fact that, in a case of small-pox occurring some time since, the remedy alluded to was efficaciously administered, before the manifestation of febrile symptoms. This circumstance seems to indicate that cream of tartar is an antidote to the variolous virus. The accuracy of this supposition appears to be confirmed by its speedy and extraordinary efficacy in cases where the poison has exerted a terrible influence throughout the system. Considerations of a scientific character point to the same conclusion. Should the supposition be a correct one, the important question would then arise, whether cream of tartar administered to persons exposed to small-pox infection might not prove an invaluable prophylactic. An incident indicative of this is to be found in the remarkable exemption from small-pox in the wine-producing districts of France.

Allow me, my Lords, most respectfully to beg your especial attention to the inestimable value of my late father's specific in the earlier stages of small-pox. When administered at this period, the fever is in two or three hours subdued, the eruption arrested, and suppuration intercepted. Your Lordships will at once perceive the great importance of thus, in a great degree, if not entirely, preventing the propagation of the disease, and wholly avoiding disfigurement. The details of a number of cases, illustrative of the truth of these assertions, are in my possession, and should your Lordships desire me to do so, I will transmit them to your Most Honorable Council with the names and addresses of the parties.

I have much pleasure in enclosing for your Lordships' perusal, a certificate as to his observation of my late father's remedy, given by T. Napper, Esq., a member of the medical profession, and long a resident in this town.

I respectfully beg that your Most Honorable Council would be pleased to order an investigation to be made, as to the prophylactic virtues of cream of tartar in regard to small-pox infection, and that the efficacy of this remedial agent may be thoroughly tested, antecedently to, and at the commencement of the eruptive stage of the variolous disease.

Most respectfully soliciting your Lordships' acquiescence in the publication of the correspondence on this subject, I beg to subscribe myself, your Lordships' obedient servant, CHARLES ROSE.

The Right Honorable the Lords of her Majesty's Privy Council.

The following is the certificate generously and disinterestedly given by Mr. Napper:

DORKING, May 12th, 1863.

I hereby certify that, while many years one of the medical officers of the Dorking Union, I had numerous opportunities of observing the very remarkable efficacy of the late Mr. Thomas Rose's remedy for small-pox. Particularly among the poor the remedy was a most popular one, but at the time referred to I was not acquainted with its nature, though astonished at its extraordinary success. THOMAS NAPPER, M. R. C. S., Etc.

A communication, as follows, was received from the Medical Officer of the Privy Council, in reply to that addressed to their Lordships on the 26th of May:

MEDICAL DEPARTMENT OF THE PRIVY COUNCIL OFFICE,
May 29th, 1863.

SIR—I am directed by the Lords of her Majesty's Council to acknowledge the receipt of your letter of May 20th, and to say that their Lordships will deal with this letter as they dealt with your communication of May 4th.

With regard to your publishing the correspondence which you have had with their Lordships, my Lords have no opinion to express..

I am, sir, your obedient servant,

JOHN SIMON.

Other correspondence with the resident surgeon of the small-pox hospital has since taken place. The publication of it is postponed, at least, for the present.

On the 8th of June the writer, acting on the advice of a medical gentleman long engaged in professional duties in India, addressed a letter to Sir Charles Wood, Bart., her Majesty's Secretary of State for that dependency,

In this communication a reference was made to "the inestimable value of so efficacious and innocuous a remedy, to a country suffering from small-pox so much as India; a remedy not opposed to the predilections of caste, nor affected by the temperature of climate." An allusion was made, in the letter referred to, to the probable preventive properties of the bi-tartrate, and a request preferred, in conclusion, that Sir C. Wood might "direct the transmission of this invaluable remedy to India, and that its curative and prophylactic virtues may be there tested."

A reply to this communication, dated July 4th, acknowledged its receipt, and informed the writer "that as the remedy in question does not appear to have undergone the test of any extended trial by public authorities in this country, Sir Charles Wood must decline to comply with your request."

It will hardly be irrevelent to add that, during the sheep small-pox epidemic, prevailing some months ago, the attention of three or four large flock-masters in the West of England was directed to the bi-tartrate as a probable remedy. If, as some writers maintain, ovine variola is identical in nature with human, there is every reason to believe that the specific for small-pox in man, would be equally remedial for the disease among sheep. The question is the more pressing just now, seeing that by a recent Government announcement, the practice of sheep inoculation increases the mortality from the disease, and that the experiments lately made with vaccination have proved "very unsatisfactory." The subject is surely one of sufficient importance to justify a trial of the bi-tartrate, both as a cure and a preventive. Should it be unsuccessful, little harm will result from the experiment, but if successful a great advantage would be gained for the grazier and the country.

"Facts," says and old but true proverb, "are stubborn things." Living proofs of the efficacy of a remedy are the best evidences of its virtues. Theory may be good, as an incentive to experiment, but fact, as a proof of its correctness, is better. More than thirty years have elapsed since the large majotity of the multitudinous cases referred to occurred. Comparatively few of the late years have been treated by the specific; enough, however, to show that, while the dreaded and loathsome disease remains the same, the remedy, "safe, speedy, and certain," is equally efficacious to prevent its development and to cure it in its most virulent form. The great value of the specific in at once arresting the progress of the disease, and the importance of its early administration, cannot be too emphatically insisted upon. Small-dox has its gradations of development. To stay its its progress in the earliest stage possible, is the dictate of wisdom. If the virus can be antidoted before producing its mischievous effects, so much the better. To adopt effectual remedial measures in the fever stage, is to intercept the eruption. To pursue the same course at the commencement of the eruptive, prevents suppuration.

In most of the cases about to be detailed, rhubarb was administered in conjunction with cream of tartar; in others, the bi-tartrate alone. The names and addresses of the patients whose initials only are given, are in the possession of the writer.

The case of Mrs. Batchelor, of Stone Bridge, Dorking, is a remarkable one:

In May, 1856, three of her children (whose cases will be presently detailed) had been suffering from small-pox, a fourth was failing, and a neighbor's family was then under the influence of the disease. Mrs. Batchelor herself was seized with the premonitory symptoms of the small-pox, aching of the head and bones, general languor and discomfort. The fever stage, however, had not yet set in, for, to use her own words, she "had no eruption, no redness of the skin, was not hot, but felt very unwell, in fact, quite ill." The late Mr. Rose saw her, when in this condition, and with his great experience in variola, at once pronounced the case to be one of small-pox. Mrs. Batchelor took one dose only of the remedy, was speedily better, and in a few hours after was perfectly well. Her infant, who was also evidently failing at the same time, was cured by the medicine taken by its mother.

Mrs. Batchelor had been three times vaccinated: in infancy, and when seven and twelve years of age.

The following cases are illustrative of the efficacy of the remedy in the febrile stage:

Wallace Batchelor, about eight years old, son of the last-named patient, was suffering from small-pox simultaneously with his mother. "Had great redness of the skin, but no pimples." Took a quarter of a pint of the medicine at ten in the morning, was relieved in about two hours, and played about the house. "The redness of the skin had all disappeared by the evening, and the next day he was out at play, as if nothing had been the matter." The patient had been vaccinated.

Michael Croly, a lodger's child, residing in the same house, was similarly attacked, and took the remedy at the same time as the previous patient. Was also relieved in about two hours, and played about in-doors in the afternoon." The next day, was out of doors, apparently as well as usual. Had been vaccinated about two months before.

The subjoined recent cases show the effect of the remedy in smaller doses:

Mr. King, a basket-maker, residing at Leslie Park road, Croydon Common, had a severe attack of small-pox in April last, and was professionally treated.

On Saturday, May 9th, a daughter, in her seventh year, was evidently failing with the disease. On that day and the following, the usual symptoms were developed. On Monday the eruption appeared, and toward the evening of the same day, had assumed a pustular form. Half a wine-glassful of the remedy was administered at 8 p.m., and a quarter of a winé-glassful only, three hours afterwards. The diminished dose was continuously repeated. The fever had evidently abated after the third dose—or when a wine-glassful of the medicine had been taken. The eruption, the following morning, had considerably increased, but a marked difference was observable in that appearing after the fourth dose. The modified eruption was "weaker and watery." On Wednesday the eruption generally was dying away. The administration of the medicine was discontinued on Saturday, when the child was "quite well." She had been vaccinated in infancy. An interesting and highly important feature in connection with this case is, that the modified eruption had completely gone within a week after its first appearance. The pustular eruption still remained, but was then "fading fast." It is equally worthy of remark that a slight pitting has resulted from the primary eruption. The facts of this case, and the experience in others, plainly indicate the necessity of a larger dose. Had this been given, it is more than probable that the modified eruption would never have appeared. The interesting result however, has amply justified the experiment.

Two more cases afterwards occurred in the same family:

On the following Monday (May 18th), a son ten years of age was attacked. A wine-glassful of the remedy was administered at 9 a. m., and the fever abated in two hours. A second dose was given six hours afterwards, when "the fever quite left him." "Three red spots of a hard substance, not watery," afterwards came out. On Wednesday he was "busily at play, as though nothing had been the matter with him." The eruption was "clean gone within a week." The patient had been vaccinated.

In this case had the dose been repeated in three, instead of six hours, or had a larger quantity—as in a previously reported case*—been given, even a popular eruption might have been prevented.

Another daughter, in her sixth year, was attacked simultaneously with her brother. Half a wine-glassful of the remedy was given at 4 p. m., on the same day, and repeated in six hours. The eruption in this case was of the same character as in the preceding one, but more copious. On Wednesday the fever had quite left her. As in the previous case, the eruption had entirely disappeared in a week. This patient had not been vaccinated.

The necessity of a larger dose, or a more frequent repetition, in this case, as in the others, is evident. The escape from an attack by other members of the family, is attributed to taking the bi-tartrate as a preventive.

A married daughter of Mr. King's and her child, afterwards failed with small-pox, "took the medicine," and had the disease "very light." "They are neither of them pitted, for they had scarce any spots."

The three following cases are those of other children of a patient already referred to. They occurred a few days previous to her's:

Alfred Batchelor, five years of age, was taken as with a billious attack, was very hot, head swollen. He continued in this state for two or three days, during which he was in bed. About the third day an eruption appeared on his face A quarter of a pint dose of the remedy was administered, and in little more than two hours an improvement had taken place. The fever had diminished and the patient "looked brighter." In the afternoon of the same day he played about in-doors with the other children, and on the following day, was out at play as usual. The eruption, excepting on that side of the head which had lain on the pillow, had quite disappeared in two or three days. This child, remarkably enough, had been vaccinated about a week. "The arm rose more after the eruption came out. He had a very fine arm. He got well of the small-pox before he did of the cow-pox!"†

Lydia Batchelor, aged thirteen, failed a few days after the last-named patient. Swollen head; was very feverish and delirious. Medicine given at noon. At this time the eruption appeared, "very thick under the skin, and some pimples were out." About three o'clock the patient came down stairs perfectly sensible, and in the evening was so far recovered as to engage in play. The next day, was out of doors, and helped her mother in household duties. Had been twice vaccinated.

William Batchelor, aged eleven, was attacked simultaneously with his sister. With the exception of delirium, symptoms similar to those of last case. The remedy administered at the same time. Relief obtained in two

* Case of Wallace Batchelor.

† The question has been appropriately asked: "If vaccination cannot neutralize a present virus, how can it neutralize at a far distant date, one which the system has not yet imbibed?" To this interrogation, the following may be added: What semblance of argument for vaccination still remains, when by the use of a remedy a patient recovers more quickly and with less suffering, from small-pox—the disease sought to be prevented—than from cow-pox—the disease inflicted as a prophylactic?

hours; the patient at play in the afternoon. Next day, appeared as well as usual. In two or three days the eruption had quite gone. Had been vaccinated. It is almost needless to add that neither this patient, nor any other member of his family, is pitted.

It is worthy of note, that a young man who played with the last two patients, on the day the specific was administered, failed with small-pox a fortnight afterwards, at Red Hill (and not taking the remedy), had it severely, and is badly pitted.

The subjoined case is remarkably illustrative of the efficacy of the specific in an early stage. It occurred in the spring of 1856:

Thomas Redford, aged 23, a carman, then and now residing at Dorking, was seized with the premonitory symptoms of small-pox. He was very unwell for two days, and on the third day the eruption appeared on the forehead, where his hat had pressed. Half a pint of the remedy was taken at 8 p. m. No more was administered afterwards. On the following morning, so great was the improvement in the patient, that he arose to breakfast and ate heartily of it. A copious eruption in its incipient stage, was plainly visible on the hands of the patient and other parts of the body, "killed"—to use his own expression—by the action of the medicine. An aperient was taken in the course of the morning. In the afternoon the patient employed himself at digging in a garden, and the next day followed his avocation of carter, as usual. He has enjoyed good health ever since. As a proof that the complaint from which the patient was suffering was really small-pox, it may be mentioned that he contracted the disorder from sleeping with his brother, who suffered severely from the disease. It is equally certain that the case was not one "modified by vaccination," for, when about 13 years of age, 16 punctures on the right arm and 12 on the left, were made, "without effect," by the vaccine lancet. This patient's wife and child, and other members of his family residing at Kingsfold, near Warnham, Sussex, were also cured by the remedy.

W. R., aged 19, residing at Dorking, failed with small-pox in the spring of 1856. The attack was so severe that the disease became confluent, and the sufferer delirious. The patient had been confined to his bed some days when the specific was first taken. A bottle of hot water was applied to his feet, in conjunction with the administration of the remedy. The patient became sensible in little more than an hour, and his improvement was so rapid that in a few days after he walked a distance of several miles. He is but little pitted. He had been vaccinated in childhood; three cicatrices perfect.

Mrs. Worsfold, aged about 55, of the Surrey Yeoman Inn, Dorking, an aunt of the preceding patient, failed with the small-pox nearly at the same time. The remedy was taken soon after the eruption appeared, and the patient was speedily relieved.

A friend residing in one of the home counties wrote, after describing a case of. small-pox, in March last:—

"Our third little boy had the same symptoms, followed in three or four days by a considerable eruption. The doctor pronounced it a case of small-pox. With some difficulty the cream of tartar was given. We could only administer about half a wine-glassful at the time, but its effects were apparent in removing the angry appearance of the pustules, and in preventing suffering. The doctor told me he should have regarded it as a case modified by vaccination. The little fellow has never been vaccinated."

The same correspondent, in a subsequent letter, wrote:—

"Our servant has also had the disease. Her's was a remarkable case. Two half-pint doses of the remedy were administered, and she had not the least trace of the eruption a week after it appeared."

He wrote also, in another letter:—

"Our minister called on Monday evening, saying, his two little boys after being poorly, had an eruption, similar to our boy. I gave him the remedy, and it was taken. The next day they were much better, and the following, nearly all traces had disappeared."

The subjoined cases demonstrate the remedial virtues of the specific, at a more advanced stage:—

John Ayliffe,* of Effingham, near Dorking, failed with small-pox, in March, 1855. The eruption appeared after the usual premonitory symptoms. It was not till two days had elapsed that the remedy was administered. A half-pint dose was given between six and seven in the evening, the patient being then in bed. He felt better in three quarters of an hour, got up and kept about till his usual bed-time. On the following day, the patient had still further improved, and on the day succeeding this, the eruption began to die away. Two or three almost imperceptible "pits" on the face, are all the traces of the disease now remaining.

T. R., aged 25, residing in a village near Dorking, was vaccinated in May, 1860, and a week afterwards failed with small-pox. The eruption had been pustular some days when the medicine was given. A half-pint dose of the medicine was taken by the patient one evening. The next day he was considerably better, and able to get out of doors. He got well rapidly from that time, without more medicine.

H. R., aged 18, was vaccinated at the same time as his brother, and failed with small-pox a day earlier. Had the disease very bad. "Was unable to turn in bed without help." Took a half-pint dose of the remedy, the same evening as the previous patient. The next day "was able to walk in the garden." Took another dose only, in the afternoon of that day, and continued to improve rapidly till well.

A young man, a neighbor of the last two patients, failed with small-pox about the same time, and was cured by taking a half-pint dose of the medicine when the eruption was coming out.

Peter Hamshere, aged 33, residing at West Horsley, near Guildford, has been very recently cured by the remedy. Early in the present month (July), he was seized with the premonitory symptoms of small-pox—aching of the bones and cold shivers. These symptoms continued several days. On Friday, the 10th, the eruption appeared, and on Sunday, the 12th, had become pustular. A half-pint dose was administered about noon on the last-named day, and a second dose at five o'clock. He was considerably better in the evening, and the next morning felt able to work, and on the following resumed his usual employment.

Enough cases have been already detailed to show the specifical properties of the bi-tartrate in the earlier stages of small-pox. Others of a more severe and hopeless nature remain to be given. Many cases of this description, treated by the late Mr. Rose, in the years immediately succeeding his discovery, might be narrated. A preference of selection however, has been given to more recent cases, not because the remote ones were less illustrative of the remedial efficacy of the specific, but from the fact that the recent generally possess greater interest, and may be more easily confirmed or refuted.

The case of George Baker,† a little boy residing at West street, Dorking, was an extremely desperate one. Seized with small-pox about Michaelmas, 1847, the disease progressed till all hope had gone. The patient was blind and insen-

* The terribly severe case of this patient's brother is described in a letter, on p. 24.

† The father of this patient, who recently narrated the case to the writer, is now living at Cape Place, Dorking.

sible, and lay utterly prostrate and apparently lifeless. It was thought at one time, indeed, that he was dead. While in this state as much of the remedy was given as could be. An hour and a half after its first administration the patient moved an eye. He gradually improved from that time till he perfectly recovered. The mother, and a brother of this patient, who severely suffered from the disease, and three other members of the family, were also cured by the medicine. One poor child had already died before the remedy was resorted to.

The case of Joseph Peters,* a young man, was a severe and well-nigh hopeless one. The disease had become confluent, and the patient delirious. He was sensible about two hours after the administration of the medicine, and got better from that time. This patient had been vaccinated, without effect, in childhood. He attributes his escape from death solely to taking the remedy. The case occurred in 1850. A child of the patient's, and other relatives, were cured about the same time.

G. C., a carpenter of middle age. A very bad case of confluent small-pox; occurring in 1849. The patient delirious, livid, "given over." Relieved in about two hours by a half-pint dose of the remedy. and ultimately got well.

Mrs. Kempshall,† Edward-street, Kingsland-road, London, failed with the small-pox in the spring of 1856. She grew continually worse, till the disease had become confluent. Her head was much swollen. She was blind and delirious. A friend of the patient's at Dorking, hearing of her dangerous condition, obtained the remedy, and visited her. A half-pint dose was administered between 9 and 10 p. m. The patient soon became sensible, and by four o'clock the next morning could see. She got better from that time.

Another female and her three children, residing in the same house as the last mentioned patient, were attacked with the disease, took the remedy early, and were soon well.

Mr. Philip Muggeridge, of Manor Farm, Abinger, near Dorking, in a letter dated June 12th last, relative to his being cured of small-pox by the remedy, writes:

"My friends thought I should never recover, and hearing of Mr. Rose, sent for him. He came, and gave me some of his medicine. I drank about one quart. My head was very much swollen, and I was very full of the pock all over. I was at a burning heat, and very thirsty. I was in bed: he made me get up, and come down stairs; and in one hour after I had taken his mixture‡ the fever had left me. I was in no pain after, and got about directly. You can make use of my name if you like to do so. I am sure everyone ought to know such a valuable medicine."

The following letter from a mechanic, conclusively attests the beneficial effect of the specific, in a desperately hopeless case. The patient had been vaccinated:

DEPTFORD, June 14th, 1863.

SIR: I received your letter this week, and I feel a pleasure in answering it, respecting the cure of myself. I was taken ill with the small-pox March 6th, 1855. When the eruption came out I was taken to bed and a doctor sent for. He attended me six days. The seventh day he came, he gave no hope of my ever recovering. He told my friends it was impossible for me to live through the night. My head was swollen to twice the size it ought to have been, and my tongue swollen out of my mouth. I was totally blind for three weeks, and thought I should never see the blessed light again, but, thank God, I can see as well now as ever I could. The same evening that the doctor reported it impossi-

* This patient now resides at Cotmandene, Dorking.

† Mrs. Kempshall has since died of consumption.

‡ In this case and the succeeding one, rhubarb was administered in conjunction with the bi-tartrate. In most of the very recent cases, subsequently reported, cream of tartar only was taken.

ble for me to live through the night, one of my neighbors at Effingham* saw my sister, and said, "Why not go to Mr. Rose, at Dorking? He has done wonderful cures in small-pox." My friends sent to your father, and he sent two doses for me—one to take that evening. Then there was another trial—my friends thought me too far gone to take the medicine, and I believe my nurse gave it to me with a feather. Anyone would hardly believe how very much better I was the next day, Nearly all the fever gone from my throat, and I was able to swallow the second dose with pleasure. My throat was so much better that I could take some gruel from that time. In the course of two or three days my nurse got me up, and into the next apartment, and in less than a week I could get there myself, although I was still totally blind. I continued to get better until my health was quite restored again; and, thank God, I am not very much pitted.

I should feel most happy, sir, to tell any one who may please to enquire of me about my case, and I do most sincerely hope that you will be successful in your undertaking. If anyone should wish to see me I shall be at Leatherhead on Monday. I think most likely I shall be there for two or three months.

I am, sir, yours very respectfully,

To Mr. C. Rose. WILLIAM AYLIFFE.

P. S.—If you should please to send anyone to see me, or write, my address will be: at Mr. Lipscombe's, Builder, Leatherhead, Surrey.†

The following case is remarkably illustrative of the importance of proportioning the administration of the remedy to the severity, or otherwise, of the attack, and of combining a judicious treatment:

On Friday evening, the 19th of June last, a young married lady residing in Surry, was attacked with the premonitory symptoms of small-pox; pains in the back and head, weakness and weariness. So general was the prostration, indeed, that the patient felt almost unable to move. On the next day (Saturday), the fever had unmistakeably set in. Various cooling drinks were given without beneficial effect. The fever had increased on the succeeding day, and in the evening a few pimples were observable on one of the hands. On the following morning the eruption had considerably increased, and was now apparent on the face and other parts of the body. A teacupful of the remedy‡ was taken at one o'clock. The fever abated, and by half-past four the pulse had fallen from 100 or 110 to 80. The same dose was repeated in the course of the evening, and a change in the eruption was perceptible on the following morning (Tuesday). A mistake was now committed.§ Some porter was taken by the patient, and the fever slightly returned. Another dose of the remedy was administered in the evening, and on the following morning the febrile symptoms were completely gone. The return of the fever caused a slight increase of the eruption; this, however was of a modified character and soon disappeared. The patient's general health, preceding the attack had not been strong. The continued presence of the fever doubtlesss till further reduced her strength. The administration of the remedy was postponed two days, at least, too long. The delay arose, however, from an uncertainty as to the nature of the ailment. Notwithstanding the unfavorable circumstances referred to, the patient continued to improve from the period when the secondary fever was subdued, and had so far regained her strength on the Saturday following as then to attend to her domestic duties, and go out of doors. That the attack was one of small-pox is evident from the nature of the premonitory symptoms, from the depression which was observable in the centre of the three or four pustules arriving partially at maturity, and from a slight pitting resulting from them. Another circumstance contributory to such a conclusion

* A village near Dorking, where the case occurred.

† The brother of the patient states that the latter was totally insensible, and that his incoherent expressions were uttered in a whisper. The brother avers also, 'that the patient became sensible the same evening the specific was taken.

‡ The following were the proportions: Bi-tartrate of Potash, ¾ oz., Rhubarb, 3 grs. (this quantity was substituted by mistake for 12 grs.). water 1 pint.

§ Since writing the above it has been ascertained that a stimulant was taken on the two preceding days.

was the prevalence of small-pox, to a considerable extent, in the neighborhood. The patient had not been vaccinated. It ought not to be omitted to be stated that a youthful relative, residing in the same house, was seized with symptoms indicative of the small-pox. and was speedily relieved by the remedy.

A letter received on the 10th instant (July), from Wick, near Littlehampton, gives the following interesting details:

A young woman named Eliza Baker failed with small-pox. She was very unwell for two or three days. "Was coming out quite full" when the remedy was taken. She found great relief from it, and the eruption "quite went away." The patient began taking the medicine on the 9th of June, and in two or three days was able to do her work.

Louisa Mathews, about 12 years of age, also failed. She took the remedy on the 21st of June. The eruption "was coming out very full on the face. She took nine wineglassfuls from Saturday night to Sunday night, and found great relief from it directly she took it." The disease had been very bad in the house.

Eliza Carpenter, age about 38, felt very ill, took two wineglassfuls of the remedy and found relief directly. The next day, as she was very thirsty, she took eight wineglassfuls more, and in a day or two was quite well.

Thomas Bravery, about 60, felt very ill a day or two, and the doctor said he was failing with the small-pox. The remedy was given on the 27th of June. He took altogether about one pint, and is quite well now.

John Booker, age about 48, residing at Littlehampton, felt very ill last Sunday and Monday (July 5th and 6th), with cold chills and back-ache. He took in all about one pint. He found relief directly he took the first dose, and is quite well and at work to-day (July 9th.)

A tradesman living at Wick, suffered last month (June), so severely from small-pox as to be delirious and not expected to recover. He continued to improve after the administration of the remedy—at first by tea-spoonfuls—and five days after was "perfectly sensible and out of danger" In this case, however, the sole merit of recovery can hardly be claimed for the specific, a professional treatment of the patient being simultaneously continued. This patient's wife subsequently appeared to be failing with the disease, took the remedy and was soon better.

Another letter, received also on the 10th instant, from a lady residing at Brockham, near Dorking, states respecting two cases of small-pox recently occurring there:

The girl, who is 11 years old, was considered in a dangerous state when she first took the remedy, and from that time began to mend, and is now quite well. Mrs. W——, the mother of the girl, had symptoms of the disease coming on, so began the remedy directly, and had no other medicine, and is now well. Her husband and one boy commenced taking it at the same time, and have had no symptoms of the disease, which they attribute solely to the remedy. It is only right to add that the younger patient was under professional treatment, and that the medical gentleman in attendance, with a liberality highly creditable, avowed his belief in the remedial virtues of the bi-tartrate, and acquiesced in its administration.

The following recent severe case of small-pox demonstrates in the most conclusive manner, the marvelous effect of the specific:

James Freeman, aged 23, a blacksmith, residing at Effingham, near Dorking, had just returned from militia service at Guildford, where small-pox at the time he left that town was prevailing. On Friday, the 5th of last month (June), he felt somewhat unwell. The next day (Saturday) the patient was still more indisposed. He had violent pains, particularly in his head and shoulders, as from a bilious attack. Fever now set in, and about noon on the following day (Sunday) an eruption appeared. On Monday he was too ill to get up. On the two following days he continued to grow worse. On Thursday afternoon he had become delirious. On Friday, the 12th, the patient's condition was highly dangerous. His appearance, too, was frightful. The disease had become confluent. The patient's head and face were so swollen that his eyes were completely hidden. The delirium had increased; he was blind; his throat was dreadfully bad; his lips were hideously swollen. The spectacle presented was pitiable in the extreme. On the same day, a neighbor, who himself had been cured, and to whom, some time before, the writer had given the formula, called and saw the patient. A pint of the remedy (¾ oz. of Cream of Tartar and 12 grs. Rhubarb) was given between seven and eight in the evening, and a second dose the same night. In about an hour after the patient had first taken the remedy, he fell into a doze. On the following morning (Saturday) he was much better; the fever had quite left him; his throat was relieved; he was sensible; could see, and was in no pain. The swelling of the head and face, though still considerable, had abated. The next day (Sunday he had much improved. He got up, dressed, sat at the bedroom window, and smoked. The day following, (Monday) he walked in the garden, and drank, without apparent injury, some porter. The two succeeding days, (Tuesday and Wednesday,) he continued to improve, and on Thursday, the 18th, i. e., within a week from the time the remedy was first taken, he was at work at the forge.

Although this patient's case was so exceedingly critical, at the time the specific was first administered, the climax (or "turn") of the disease had not yet been reached. A medical gentleman, who has since seen, and interrogated him, expresses a decided opinion, that "under God, the patient owes his life to the remedy," as "had he not taken it, he must have died." The marked success, resulting in this instance from the administration of an unusually large quantity, is another illustration of the importance, if not the absolute necessity, of large doses in severe cases. The patient was vaccinated when five years of age, the cicatrices on both arms being still perfect. Notwithstanding the severity of the case, he will be but little, if at all marked.

The writer has much pleasure in inserting the following letter, received just before going to press, from G. K. Paxon, Esquire, a highly respectable medical practitioner, residing at Dorking. The important testimony to the remedial virtues of the bi-tartrate, so kindly and liberally given by Mr. Paxon, is the more valuable and interesting, from its referring to cases which have recently occurred, within the range of that gentleman's own professional practice:

"DORKING, SURREY, July 21st, 1863.

Dear Sir,

I beg to inform you that I have given the bi-tartrate of potash in three cases of small-pox—two occurring lately, about five miles from here—and one a year ago.

In two cases advanced to the postular stage of the disease, it had the immediate effect of subduing the fever, dispelling the swelling of the head and face, and arresting the supperation of the postules—thereby preventing the disfigurement of 'pitting.'

In the third case, (consequent upon one of the former,) the eruptive stage—which was severe—speedily subsided into a scanty and scattered crop of minute postules, appearing one day, and becoming shriveled and decaying in the next.

Expressions of great relief followed the exhibition of the medicine and convalescence was rapid.

These cases, insignificant, perhaps, in themselves, go far to confirm the success of the treatment of variola, so fully described by you in so many instances; and my faith in its efficacy is such, that I should administer it in every case of small-pox that I may be called upon to treat.

I remain, dear Sir,

Yours very truly,

GEO. K. PAXON."

Mr. Chas. Rose.

With such an amount of evidence as that presented, the impartial and ingenuous inquirer after truth, will have but little hesitation as to a decision. The varied and numerous cases narrated, confirmed by a multitude of others, conclusively demonstrate that, for the fever of small-pox, the Bi-tartrate of Potash is an invaluable specific, and that, in all stages of the disease, its remedial virtues are uniformly efficacious. Should anyone, especially any member of the profession, be still sceptical, let him test the remedy on the first opportunity, and for the sake of humanity announce the result.

A perusal of the cases reported will have suggested that, judgment as to the administration of the remedy, and the treatment of the patient, must at all times be exercised. The severity of the attack, the age, mode of life, and constitution of the patient should each be considered. Under ordinary circumstances, and particularly in the earliest stage, the information conveyed in this pamphlet will be found amply sufficient. It is possible however, that cases of a complicated and difficult nature may arise—as they have arisen—demanding all the skill and experience obtainable. Amateur practice would then be unwise, and might be disastrous.

The great importance of an early administration has been already insisted upon. The discovery that, by promptly adopting remedial measures, the progress of the disease is effectually stayed, is scarcely second in value to that of the specific itself.

Unlike many other medicinal agents, the cure for small-pox is neither dangerous nor injurious. Its very simplicity—a recommendation rather than otherwise—has been, in fact, the greatest obstacle to its adoption; its household familiarity the cause of its depreciation.

Doubtless, were the specific a novel product of distant shores, discovered by one eminent in science, or high in social position, a different reception, than that hitherto awarded, would have awaited it. The origin of a discovery however, does not affect its value, nor its treatment its importance. Prejudice may spurn, at first, a gift so common; interest, vested and selfish, may denounce it, yet these, strong though they be, must yield to truth. Resistance to fact is as futile as it is foolish. Opposition to good is more—it is criminal.

Whether welcome or despised, the truth is now patent to the world, that *"A safe, speedy, and certain cure" for small-pox has been discovered, and that this hitherto dreaded, disfiguring, and fatal disease, by the blessing of Heaven, need be so no longer.*

THE DISCOVERY OF VACCINATION.

Dr. Huillet, medical officer in charge at Pondicherry, has availed himself of a sojourn there to verify the truth as to whether vaccination was practised in India in very remote periods, and he has found the mention of variola and cow-pox in a work, attributed to Dharwantari, who lived many years before Hippocrates. William Bruce, consul at Bushira, believes that vaccination was for a long time practised in Persia, and Humbolt says that for a number of years the inhabitants of the Cordilleras had noticed the preservative effects of vaccine. Without doubt the ancient author of Sataya Grantham is entitled to priority, but it was a Frenchman, Rabaut Ponniner, brother to Rabaut St. Etienne, Protestant minister at Massilargues, near Lunel, who discovered in 1784 that inoculation from the teat of a cow was a preventive against small-pox. He communicated his idea to two Englishmen, Ireland and Pugh, who spoke of it to Jenner. Mr. Ireland subsequently wrote to M. Rabaut, who, according to the *Journal de Therapeutique*, for May, 1877, declared himself satisfied.—*Medical Press.*

VIRUS AND SMALL-POX.

HOW THE FIRST IS MADE—IS IT WORSE THAN THE SECOND—WHAT THE EVOLUTIONISTS SAY OF VACCINATION.

As so much of the best blood, and the worst blood, too, of Detroit is now mingled with what is called pure bovine virus, the public may be interested in learning what the virus is and how it is prepared. It all comes from Dr. Pettet's institution in Cleveland. Dr. Pettet's laboratory is simply a cow stable. The raw material is represented by a number of yearling thoroughbred heifers. Young and blooded stock are used on account of the thinness of their skin and the purity of their blood from all disease, and preference is given to the females on account of their having a large surface of hairless skin on their udders, which is peculiarly convenient. The udders and the insides of the thighs of a heifer are shaved clean of stray hairs, carefully scarified all over and then annointed with fresh vaccine taken on the spot from a previously diseased animal. In ten days time all the annointed surface has festered and become covered with pustules. At this time the first crop of vaccine is taken. The heifer is laid on her back. The postules are tapped, and, in the amber colored liquor flowing therefrom are dipped the so-called "points" and "quills" of commerce. The points are thin slips of ivory about the size of a small penknife blade, The quills are common goosequills. To these points and quills the gummy liquor sticks, growing hard on being dried. These points and quills retail for twenty-five cents, and are good each for two or three vaccinations. At the end of three weeks the festers have gone down and the scabs have formed over the whole surface which had previously been inoculated. These are removed and cut up into little squares of about a quarter of an inch in size and three grains in weight. They are then placed on squares of black wax, to which they adhere tightly, are thoroughly dried and wrapped, first in cotton batting and afterwards in rubber cloth. They thus retail for three dollars apiece, or a dollar a grain. Great care is taken of the vaccine in all forms to prevent exposure to cold under 40 degrees, or heat over 80 degrees, or the least moisture, any of which conditions would destroy the virtue of the virus. Even with all this precaution vaccine becomes useless after it is two or three weeks old, and should always be used before it is a week old. Old virus, or virus in the least decomposed, is poisonous, and may prove fatal to the person inoculated with it. It is owing to the fact that large quantities of it grow old on the producers' hands, as well as the expense of buying and hiring valuable stock, that makes the pure bovine virus so dear in the market.

This is the manner in which "pure bovine virus" is produced, and at the very best one can hardly help thinking that "pure" is not just the right word in the right place. It is hardly to be wondered at that many people and many of the profession at first resisted the practice of a process which is inherently so unclean, and is associated in every step with disease and corruption. Its use having become almost universal, the profession and people generally ascribe to it the decadence of the more horrible disease it is designed to prevent, and they have at least the coincidence to sustain them. Still, murmurs are beginning to be heard, and from very high quarters too, against the whole system, and there are men of the highest scientific attainments who maintain that vaccination has had very little, if anything, to do with the decadence of small-pox, and is of no use to-day as a preventive. From the modern doctrine of evolution, the opponents of vaccination derive the theory that small-pox itself has caused its own decay by killing off the individuals and families most susceptible to it. Each epidemic visitation has been less wide-spread and has found fewer victims, until now there are only left isolated individuals here and there who incur any danger of taking it. It has literally devoured its inheritance of human victims, is starved out, and is now no more dangerous than any other disease. They who believe in this theory regard vaccination as an unmitigated evil, and as the frequent cause of innumerable diseases, and advise to avoid it as one would small-pox itself.

The reader can take his choice between the schools.

Spotted something that isn't quite right?

Let us know and we'll fix it for future reprints. And as a thank you for your diligence, we'll send you a free Sothis book of your choice.

publisher@sothis.press

This page intentionally left blank

Made in the USA
Monee, IL
08 November 2026

68102151R00023